MEDICAL TERMINOLOGY

*The Best and Most Effective Way
to Memorize, Pronounce and
Understand Medical Terms*

Workbook

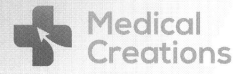

Medical Creations

Contents

INTRODUCTION

A good grounding in medical terminology is absolutely essential to succeed in any of the medical and health-related fields. Medical terminology facilitates medical communication, which in turn is the underlying framework for the discovery, dissemination and propagation of medical knowledge.

Medical students and professionals understand this. Hence, the immense popularity of our medical terminology textbook **Medical Terminology: The Best and Most Effective Way to Memorize, Pronounce and Understand Medical Terms**. The textbook is a comprehensive yet concise introduction to medical terminology. It's a must-read for those looking to hone their knowledge of medical terms.

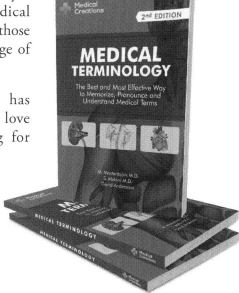

Feedback from our readers has informed us that while they love the textbook, they're looking for more quizzes and exercises on medical terminology. This workbook has been prepared to address that need. Here you'll find plenty of questions and exercises to test your knowledge and understanding of medical terms.

WAYS TO USE THE WORKBOOK

This medical terminology workbook is a companion to the textbook. As such, it can be used in the following ways:

A. After you've finished the textbook, you can use this workbook to test your knowledge retention.

B. Also, you can progress through the textbook and workbook together. Whenever you finish a chapter of the textbook, you can do the corresponding unit of exercises from the workbook. That will help you assess your knowledge retention but also serve to recapitulate the key concepts.

C. Finally, if you're feeling really confident, you can actually start off with the workbook first and see where you stand. If you find knowledge gaps, then you can go through the textbook to improve your grasp of the subject.

TIP

When doing the exercises in the workbook, remember that what's being tested is not your knowledge of medicine but how medical terms are formed.

For example, let's say there is a question, "What is inflammation of the liver called?" You might say to yourself, "How am I supposed to know that? I've never studied liver pathology." However, what you should do is focus on the principles of medical terminology—the root words and their origins.

You must've recognized the use of the word 'hepatic' for liver in different medical contexts. You might also be familiar with the quite popular convention that '-itis' stands for inflammation. So, you found your answer, "Hepatitis." You didn't need to be a medical consultant to know that!

TYPES OF EXERCISES

This medical terminology workbook contains different types of exercises. Some examples are:

- Match the columns
- Fill in the blanks
- Multiple choice questions (MCQs)
- True or false
- Label the picture

While it's clear for most exercises what needs to be done, here are instructions for some of them to remove any ambiguity.

MATCH THE COLUMNS

For such exercises, just keep in mind that the last column (the rightmost column) contains the answers that need to filled out in the 'Correct match' column.

Set A

	Clinical problem	Correct match	Prefix or suffix
5.	not working correctly or normally		itis
6.	bad		osis
7.	blood condition		pathy
8.	inflammation		mal
9.	condition or disease (usually non-inflammatory)		dys
10.	disease		emia

MCQS

Just remember that <u>only one</u> of the given answer choices is correct.

---

94. Which one of the following terms means an inflamed peritoneum?

   a.   Parotitis
   b.   Cystitis
   c.   Peritonitis
   d.   Pericarditis

TRUE OR FALSE

Put a T or F in the box next to each question according to whether you think the statement is true or false.

---

56. A subcutaneous injection is given just below the skin.

Well, that's it for now. Good luck with the exercises!

Understanding Medical Terms

EXERCISE 1 - FILL IN THE BLANKS

1. Many medical terms are a combination of a beginning, a _____ and an ending.

2. Beginnings and endings of medical terms are also called prefixes and _____

3. A _____ can be about shape, size, direction, or color.

4. A _____ can be about a test or it can describe a problem.

EXERCISE 2 - MATCH THE COLUMNS

Set A

	Clinical problem	Correct match	Prefix or suffix
5.	not working correctly or normally		itis
6.	bad		osis
7.	blood condition		pathy
8.	inflammation		mal
9.	condition or disease (usually non-inflammatory)		dys
10.	disease		emia

Set B

	Test or procedure	Correct match	Prefix or suffix
11.	ultrasonic waves		graph or graphy
12.	electricity		echo
13.	removal of		stomy
14.	picture		plasty
15.	process of taking a picture		otomy
16.	making a cut in/removing a part of		electro
17.	use of instrument for viewing		gram
18.	create an opening in		ectomy
19.	modifying the shape of/ repairing		scopy

Root Words

EXERCISE 1 - MATCH THE COLUMNS

Set A

	Root words	Correct match	Parts of the head
1.	enceph or ceph		eardrum
2.	Rhino		skull
3.	tympan or myringo		brain
4.	odont or dento		eye
5.	Crani		ear
6.	ophthalm or oculo		nose
7.	Oto		tongue
8.	Lingu		tooth

Set B

	Root words	Correct match	Muscles and bones
9.	myo		arm
10.	scapula		foot
11.	brachi or brachio		wrist
12.	carp or carpo		bones
13.	cost or costo		back
14.	dorsa		shoulder
15.	oste or osteo		rib
16.	pod or podo or ped or pedo`		muscles

EXERCISE 2 - BUILDING WORDS

Root words	Correct match	Muscles and bones
cardi or cardio	cardio	itis
Myo	echo	ology
Colo	trans	pathy
Esophag		graphy
		ostomy
		ectomy
		eal
		gram

Use the beginnings, roots and endings provided in the table above to create words that fit the definitions given below:

17. Study of the heart: _____

18. Inflammation of the heart: _____

19. Taking a picture of the heart using ultrasonic waves:

    _____

20. A picture of the heart using ultrasonic waves: _____

21. Disease of the heart muscle: _____

22. Inflammation of the colon: _____

23. Going across the esophagus: _____

24. Removal of the colon: _____

25. Creating an opening in the colon: _____

EXERCISE 3 - FILL IN THE BLANKS

Set A

26. _____ is the abnormally large upper and lower extremities brought about by an increased production of growth hormone.

27. _____ lymphadenopathy is the enlargement of diseased lymph nodes in the armpit characterized by swollen armpits.

28. Surgical repair of the eyelid is called _____.

29. _____ means anything relating to the cheek.

30. Inflammation of the skin is termed _____.

31. _____ is the backward bending of the foot or hand.

32. Gingivitis is the inflammation of the _____

33. _____ is a surgical operation to allow the surgeon to see the organs within the abdomen.

34. Bilateral means on both sides while _____ means on one side only.

35. _____ is an X-ray examination of the breasts.

Set B

36. _____ is the abnormal enlargement of breasts in males due to hormonal imbalances.

37. A nasogastric tube is introduced via the nose, through the throat and into the _____.

38. The _____ bone is a saucer-shaped bone located at the lower back area of the skull.

39. An odontoma is a benign tumor associated with the development of the _____.

40. The eye doctor (ophthalmologist) utilizes an _____ to view and check the inside of the eye.

41. _____ is an assessment method done to evaluate eyesight.

42. _____ involves the mouth as well as the pharynx.

43. Inflammation of the middle ear brought about by an infection is called _____.

44. _____ is a term used to denote a cyst which contains hair.

45. _____ is a branch of medicine which is dedicated to the care and treatment of the foot.

Set C

46. A _____ is an acoustic tool, usually placed against the chest, used for listening to the inner sounds of the body, so as to aid in diagnosis.

47. _____ is a procedure to remove fluid from the pleural space (the space between the two pleural membranes of the lung).

48. Pharmaceutical drugs used to relieve pain are called _____.

49. An element or a drug which causes the airways in the lungs to constrict and narrow is referred to as a _____.

50. A _____ is a substance, usually a chemical, which is capable of causing cancer.

51. The development of cancer is called _____.

52. _____ is an infection of the skin and its underlying tissues caused by bacteria.

53. Medical conditions affecting the arteries of the brain are categorized as _____.

54. The surgical removal of the gallbladder is called _____.

55. Surgical techniques that utilize extremely low temperatures are called _____.

EXERCISE 4 – TRUE OR FALSE

Set A

56. A subcutaneous injection is given just below the skin. ☐

57. Cyanosis of the lips is indicative of heart failure or chronic obstructive pulmonary disease. ☐

58. Cytology pertains to the study of individual organs. ☐

59. The clinical term for double vision is diplopia. ☐

60. An electroencephalogram tracks and records cardiac electrical activity. ☐

61. Infection of the stomach and the intestines, usually due to a viral or bacterial causative agent, is called gastroenteritis. ☐

62. White blood cells are also called erythrocytes. ☐

63. Esophagitis is the inflammation of the esophageal lining. ☐

64. Scar tissue overgrowth, caused by the body's exaggerated healing response is known as fibrosis. ☐

65. Excessive production of milk or milk-like discharge from the nipples is called rhinorrhea. ☐

Set B

66. Gastrostomy is a surgical procedure where an opening is created in the stomach, so that a feeding tube may be attached. □

67. A medical practice which specifically deals with female reproductive health is called gynecology. □

68. A myoma is localized pooling of blood (often solidified), brought about by bleeding from a vessel that has ruptured. □

69. Enlargement of the liver is termed splenomegaly. □

70. Heterochromia refers to a congenital condition where there is a difference in the color of the skin, the hair, but most often in the iris (e.g., one eye is brown and the other is blue). □

71. The medical term for excessive sweating is hyperthermia. □

72. Cytology refers to the scientific study of tissues. □

73. Hydrocele is a condition where the space around the testes is filled with fluid. □

74. Hysterectomy is the operative removal of the ovary for a therapeutic cause. □

75. Clinical problems that arise from medical treatment are termed iatrogenic. □

Set C

76. Jejunostomy is a surgical procedure where an opening is created through the wall of the duodenum, so that a plastic tube may be inserted for feeding.

77. Laryngitis means an inflamed larynx.

78. Leukemia is the excessive propagation of immature white blood cells, which leads to the failure of vital body organs.

79. Lithotomy is the surgical removal of tumors from areas of the urinary tract.

80. Lymphangiography is a diagnostic procedure that helps to visualize the lymphatic system.

81. Melanocytes are cells that form keratin.

82. Menorrhagia is abnormally disproportionate menstrual bleeding.

83. Meningitis is the inflamed and infected meninges, with bacteria or a virus as the causative agent.

84. Myalgia is the clinical term for joint pain.

85. Myringoplasty is a corrective operative procedure for the meninges.

EXERCISE 5 – MCQs

Set A

86. The root of a medical term usually refers to which one of the following?

   a. Medical device
   b. Body part
   c. Treatment
   d. Clinical specialty

87. A newborn baby, less than four months is called a:

   a. Infant
   b. Toddler
   c. Neonate
   d. Child

88. Which one of the following terms means the death of tissue cells?

   a. Apoptosis
   b. Necrosis
   c. Fibrosis
   d. Cellulitis

89. Surgical removal of the ovaries is known as:

   a. Hysterectomy
   b. Salpingectomy
   c. Appendectomy
   d. Oophorectomy

90. Which one of the following refers to inflamed testes accompanied by high temperature, severe pain, and swelling around the area?

    a. Prostatitis
    b. Cystitis
    c. Orchitis
    d. Cellulitis

91. Osteomyelitis is an infection, usually of bacterial origin, of which one of the following anatomical structures?

    a. Muscle
    b. Cartilage
    c. Pancreas
    d. Bone

92. The surgical reconstruction of a cleft palate is called:

    a. Septoplasty
    b. Uvuloplasty
    c. Palatoplasty
    d. Myringoplasty

93. Which one of the following means causative agent of a disease, usually a microorganism?

    a. Allergen
    b. Carcinogen
    c. Teratogen
    d. Pathogen

94. Which one of the following terms means an inflamed peritoneum?

    a. Parotitis
    b. Cystitis
    c. Peritonitis
    d. Pericarditis

95. Which one of the following terms pertains to the way the body reacts to, synthesizes, and benefits from a pharmaceutical substance?

    a. Pharmacodynamics
    b. Pharmacokinetics
    c. Pharmacotherapeutics
    d. Pharmacotherapy

Set B

96. An inflamed pharynx usually due to a viral or bacterial pathogen is known as:

    a. Pharyngeal carcinoma
    b. Laryngitis
    c. Dysphagia
    d. Pharyngitis

97. Phlebitis is the clinical term for inflammation of a:

    a. Vein
    b. Artery
    c. Capillary
    d. Lymph vessel

98. The nerve which supplies the diaphragm is appropriately called the:

    a. Tympanic nerve
    b. Vagus nerve
    c. Phrenic nerve
    d. Thoracic nerve

99. Which one of the following denotes a potentially fatal condition where air leaks into the pleural cavity?

    a. Thoracentesis
    b. Pleurisy
    c. Pneumonia
    d. Pneumothorax

100. Poliomyelitis is caused by a:

    a. Fungus
    b. Virus
    c. Bacterium
    d. Protozoan

101. An inflamed rectum commonly accompanied by pain, bleeding, and pus is called:

    a. Proctitis
    b. Colitis
    c. Empyema
    d. Hemorrhoids

102. Pyelonephritis refers specifically to a condition that affects which one of the following structures?

    a. Pelvis
    b. Kidney
    c. Bladder
    d. Adrenal gland

103. Which one of the following is a deadly condition where there is fast propagation of bacteria which release toxins into the bloodstream?

    a. Anemia
    b. Leukemia
    c. Septicemia
    d. Leukopenia

104. Which one of the following terms refers to an overly active spleen?

    a. Splenomegaly
    b. Hypersplenism
    c. Hepatomegaly
    d. Hyperthyroidism

105. Tendinitis means inflammation of which one of the following structures?

    a. Ligament
    b. Capsule
    c. Tendon
    d. Fascia

EXERCISE 6 - LABEL THE PICTURE

Use the common directional terms provided in the table below to label the picture.

Proximal	Distal	Medial	Lateral
Ventral	Dorsal	Cranial	Caudal

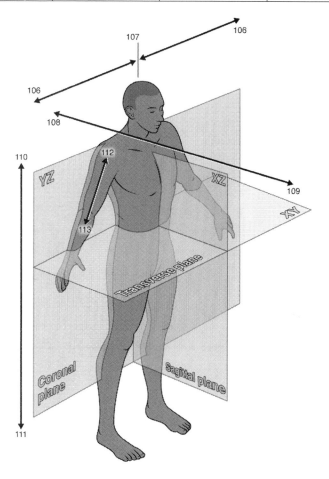

106. _____   110. _____

107. _____   111. _____

108. _____   112. _____

109. _____   113. _____

EXERCISE 7 - CROSSWORD

Down

114. Surgical removal of the tonsils
115. Muscle
117. An emergency procedure to create an opening in the windpipe in case of upper airway obstruction
119. Fat
121. Blue

ACROSS

116. Recording temperature patterns of the skin's surface in the form of images
118. Back
120. Diagnostic test assessing urine characteristics
122. Below normal thyroid hormone production
123. Blood

Pronouncing Medical Terms

EXERCISE 1 - MATCH THE COLUMNS

	Beginning with	Example	Correct match	Pronounced as
1.	cho	cholesterol		n
2.	sk	skeletal		z
3.	gy	gynecologist		j
4.	kn	knee		siy
5.	x	xerophthalmia		sk
6.	g	granuloma		si
7.	ph	physiotherapy		guh
8.	ce/ci	celiac		k
9.	gi/ge	giardiasis		f
10.	psy	psychology		guy

EXERCISE 2 - MCQs

For each word, choose the correct pronunciation of the highlighted part.

11. _Z_ika virus

    a.   ch
    b.   z
    c.   silent

12. _Sc_oliosis

    a.   k
    b.   s
    c.   sk

13. Laryn_ge_al

    a.   g
    b.   j
    c.   n

14. _Thy_roid

    a.   thi
    b.   di
    c.   fi

15. _Ty_phoid

    a.   ti
    b.   di
    c.   thy

16. _J_aundice

    a.   g
    b.   j
    c.   ch

17. _Cu_shing's syndrome

    a.   s
    b.   k
    c.   ch

Prefixes and Suffixes

EXERCISE 1 - MATCH THE COLUMNS

Set A

	Meaning	Correct match	Prefix
1.	self		hemi
2.	along with		hyp/hypo
3.	without, devoid of, not		alb
4.	external, beyond		co/con/com
5.	lacking, situated below or underneath		hyper
6.	white		a
7.	extreme, excessive, situated above		bi
8.	half		de
9.	down, to rid of		auto
10.	both, dual, twice		extra/extro

Set B

	Meaning	Correct match	Prefix
11.	small		post
12.	half		trans
13.	singular, isolated		ultra
14.	succeeding, after, located behind		syn
15.	inside, into		macro
16.	extreme, beyond normal		pre
17.	from side to side, through		idio
18.	prior, former, before, situated in front of		semi
19.	linked		micro
20.	large		intra

EXERCISE 2 - MEDICAL ANTONYMS

	Word	Meaning	Antonym
21.	Abduction	A movement away from the body's midline	
22.	Bradypnea	Abnormally slow breathing, usually under 12 breaths per minute	
23.	Endogenous depression	Biologically based depression, not caused by external factors	
24.	Euthymia	A mood that is normal and rationally positive	
25.	Hypoplasia	Under-development or incomplete development of a tissue or organ	
26.	Retrograde amnesia	Type of memory loss where the person can no longer access events that happened in the past, specifically ones before the occurrence of an injury or disease	

27

EXERCISE 3 - MEDICAL SYNONYMS

Fill in the blanks in the following table.

	Body part	Greek	Latin
27.		Odont/Odonto	Dent/Dento
28.	Kidneys		Ren/Reno
29.	Breast		Mamm/Mammo/ Mamma
30.	Navel	Omphalo	

EXERCISE 4 - SYNONYMOUS PREFIXES: PICK THE ODD ONE OUT

In this exercise, each statement is followed by a set of synonymous prefixes. Choose the option that does NOT belong to the group.

31. Bad, faulty, difficult, or painful:

   a. Dys
   b. Mal
   c. Eu

32. Against:

   a. Anti
   b. Hyper
   c. Contra

33. Above:

   a. Tachy
   b. Epi
   c. Supra

34. Under:

   a. Hypo
   b. Alb
   c. Sub

EXERCISE 5 - MCQs

Set A

35. It's called circumcision because:

    a.   The foreskin concealing the tip of the penis is removed

    b.   A circumferential incision is made around the penis's tip

    c.   It's often done for hygienic or religious reasons

36. It's called diathermy because:

    a.   High frequency electric current is used

    b.   It boosts blood flow to the treated area

    c.   It causes body tissues to be heated through

37. It's called intravascular fluid because:

    a.   It consists primarily of serum, in which blood cells are suspended

    b.   It's the fluid contained within blood vessels

    c.   It provides nutrition to the vessels

38. It's called preoperative testing because:

    a.   It's done before the surgery

    b.   It's done during the surgery

    c.   It's done after the surgery

39. It's called regurgitation because:

    a.   There is backward flow of undigested food matter back into the esophagus or the mouth

    b.   It leads to sufficient chewing and breakdown of food

    c.   It is necessary for healthy digestion

Set B

40. Which one of the following is a procedure to obtain a fluid sample from the amniotic sac?

    a. Thoracentesis
    b. Chorionic villus sampling (CVS)
    c. Amniocentesis
    d. Pleural tap

41. Which one of the following is a corrective procedure in which a bone is intentionally fractured by the surgeon in order to repair a deformity?

    a. Osteogenesis
    b. Osteomyelitis
    c. Osteoma
    d. Osteoclasis

42. Which one of the following is a surgical procedure in which a joint is immobilized after its surface is fused with that of an adjacent bone?

    a. Arthrodesis
    b. Arthroplasty
    c. Arthritis
    d. Arthroscopy

43. The surgical removal of a diseased or toxic thyroid gland is called:

    a. Hyperthyroidism
    b. Parathyroid
    c. Thyroidectomy
    d. Tonsillectomy

44. Which one of the following means examination by X-ray or CT of vessels, carried out after the introduction of a radiopaque substance?

    a. Radiography
    b. Venography
    c. Electrocardiography
    d. Angiography

45. The device used to measure blood pressure is called:

    a. Manometer
    b. Thermometer
    c. Hypertension
    d. Sphygmomanometer

46. Which one of the following terms means the removal of a sample tissue from the body of a patient so it can be examined under a microscope?

    a. Biopsy
    b. Histology
    c. Electron microscopy
    d. Cytology

47. The clinical term for correction of nasal deformities is:

    a. Rhinoplasty
    b. Myringoplasty
    c. Arthroplasty
    d. Rhinorrhea

48. Which one of the following is a tool used to examine the ear canal and the eardrum visually?

   a. Ophthalmoscope
   b. Stethoscope
   c. Otoscope
   d. Microscope

49. Which one of the following means using a needle to gain access into a vein for the purpose of drawing blood?

   a. Venectomy
   b. Phlebotomy
   c. Venography
   d. Hemophilia

EXERCISE 6 - FILL IN THE BLANKS

Set A

50. The bel a unit used to express the relative intensity of sound. One-tenth of a bel is known as _____ .

51. The monocyte is a cell with a _____ nucleus.

52. The medical term for a woman who has had no children is

_____

53. The medical term for a woman who is in her first pregnancy is

_____

54. _____ means that all four extremities are paralyzed.

55. The _____ canals of the inner ear are crucial for balance and posture.

56. Antidepressant drugs with three atom rings in their chemical structures are called _____ antidepressants.

57. The increased thirst experienced as a symptom of diabetes is termed _____

Set B

58. _____ is the clinical term for joint pain.

59. Myasthenia gravis is a severe autoimmune neuromuscular disorder which is manifested by an unpredictable degree of _____ of the body's voluntary muscles.

60. The herniation of the bladder into the weakened vaginal wall is termed _____.

61. _____ refers to dilated lymph vessels, such as due to a blockage in the local lymphatic drainage.

62. Anemia is a clinical condition characterized by red blood cell or _____ deficiency.

63. Insomnia is a persistent condition wherein the affected individual is unable to _____.

64. _____is a parasitic infection of the filarial worm which is manifested by severe swelling of the extremities owing to lymphatic blockage.

65. Inflammation of the lining of the colon is called _____.

66. _____ is a hardened mass of feces, resembling a stone, stuck in the intestinal tract.

67. An anxiolytic is a pharmaceutical drug prescribed to relieve _____.

EXERCISE 7 - TRUE OR FALSE

Set A

68. Erythrocyte is another name for a red blood cell. □

69. Exocytosis refers to the process wherein a cell swallows up a particle like a microorganism, a foreign substance, or an old blood cell. □

70. Enuresis is the clinical term for fecal incontinence. □

71. Circumduction pertains to the circular motion of an extremity. □

72. Spasm is voluntary muscular contraction. □

73. In cholestasis, there is a blockage of bile flow from the liver to the small intestine. □

74. Aortostenosis is dilatation of the aorta. □

75. Hematuria the presence of glucose in urine. □

Set B

76. The clinical term for a disproportionate enlargement of the heart is hepatomegaly.

77. Retinoblastoma a malignant eye cancer that affects the retina.

78. The medical term for bad breath is halitosis.

79. Neuropathy is a disorder that affects the peripheral nerves, often causing weakness and numbness.

80. Excessive sensitivity to light is called phonophobia.

81. In hemiplegia, the ciliary muscle of the eye is paralyzed.

82. The clinical term for profuse bleeding is hemorrhage.

83. Diarrhea is the frequent passage of loose, watery stools.

84. Atherosclerosis is a condition in which there are fatty plaque deposits in the inner walls of the arteries, causing them to harden.

85. Granulocytopenia is a significant increase in the number of granulocytes.

EXERCISE 8 - LABEL THE PICTURE

The following table contains terms for clinical conditions that affect different organs of the body. Use them to label the picture.

Hepatitis	Bronchitis	Cholecystitis	Gastritis	Colitis
Appendicitis	Carditis	Laryngitis	Cystitis	Thyroiditis

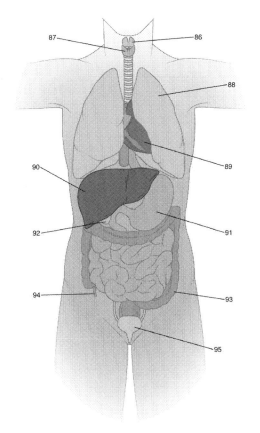

86. _____   91. _____

87. _____   92. _____

88. _____   93. _____

89. _____   94. _____

90. _____   95. _____

EXERCISE 9 - CROSSWORD

		96				97		98			
	99			100							
101											
	102										
	103										

Down

96. Smallest artery

97. Yellow-brownish to green-like fluid that the liver secretes

98. Contamination

100. To congeal or solidify fluid such as blood

ACROSS

99. 99. The ability to become erect

101. 101. Concerning therapy

102. 102. Triggers the production of collagen

103. 103. Of the ventricle

39

UNIT V

Eponyms, Homonyms and More

EXERCISE 1 - MATCH THE COLUMNS

Set A

	Definition	Correct match	Homonym
1.	A part of a bone that juts out		Epiphysis
2.	A pharmaceutical agent that triggers the action of cell molecules in a manner that they would be stimulated by the naturally occurring byproducts		Antagonist
3.	Pertaining to the mouth, its parts, and its functions		Enuresis
4.	The inability of the affected individual to pass urine		Cor
5.	The rounded edge of a long bone		Aural
6.	The midpoint		Agonist
7.	An element which neutralizes, obstructs, or combats the action of another		Apophysis
8.	Pertaining to the heart		Anuresis
9.	Pertaining to the ear, its parts, and its functions		Core
10.	Uncontrolled urination especially while sleeping at night		Oral

Set B

	Definition	Correct match	Homonym
11.	Diminished ability to comprehend speech, due to brain injury or a disease		Galacturia
12.	Milky coloring of the urine		Diastasis
13.	An individual's predisposition to a certain health condition		Dysphagia
14.	Anomalous change in the squamous epithelial cell manifested as an irregular nuclear structure; may precede the formation of a malignant neoplasm		Diaphysis
15.	Uncharacteristic flow of milk from the breasts		Dyskeratosis
16.	A condition wherein anatomical parts that are usually joined together end up separating; may occur in bones as well as muscles		Dysphasia
17.	Trouble with swallowing		Dyskaryosis
18.	Unusual keratinization (hardening of the protein in the skin, hair, and nails) which occurs in cells under the granulous layer of the epidermis		Diathesis
19.	A long bone's shaft situated between the epiphyses		Galactorrhea

Set C

	Hint	Correct match	Abbreviation
20.	Diagnosis		in vivo
21.	This is what the doctor checks for when s/he hits a tendon with a hammer		DNR
22.	A surgical procedure that is done below the knee		DVT
23.	A test performed to identify a pathogen, and to determine the best choice of medicine		LUQ
24.	In the laboratory		FX
25.	The reason why the patient sought medical attention in the first place		npo
26.	Near death patients might have such an order		DX
27.	When a blood clot occurs in a deep vein/s of the body, usually the leg		DTR
28.	An area of the abdomen		in vitro
29.	Fracture		CC
30.	An infection		C&S
31.	In the body		BKA
32.	Nothing by mouth		UTI

Set D

	Description	Correct match	Symbol
33.	At		Ø
34.	Alpha		↓
35.	Approximate		♀
36.	To Change		A
37.	Increase		<
38.	Decrease		≈
39.	Female		@
40.	Male		↑
41.	Less than		♂
42.	Greater than		Δ
43.	None		>

EXERCISE 2 – FILL IN THE BLANKS

Set A

44. The medical term concerned with body fluids is _____. (Humeral or Humoral)

45. A scientific supposition, which seeks to provide an explanation for a phenomenon is called a _____. (Hypophysis or Hypothesis)

46. The third region of the small intestine, situated between the cecum and the jejunum is known as the _____. (Ileum or Ilium)

47. _____ are ectoparasites which can infest various hair-bearing parts of the body, from the head to the toe. (Lice or Lyse)

48. The _____ is a mallet-shaped bone in the middle ear. (Malleolus or Malleus)

49. _____ refers to when a secondary malignant growth develops away from the initial site of the cancer. (Metaphysis or Metastasis)

Set B

50. _____ is a sticky secretion secreted by mucous membranes, that acts as a protectant and a lubricant. (Mucous or Mucus)

51. _____ pertains to an opening. (Osteal or Ostial)

52. _____ is to bring about the flow or the dissemination of something within a tissue. (Profuse or Perfuse)

53. _____ is the smallest subdivision in a nerve. (Radicle or Radical)

54. When part of an anatomical structure or organ is surgically removed, it is called a _____. (Resection or Recession)

55. _____ refers to the bladder. (Vesicle or Vesical)

56. _____ means viscid, gelatinous, and is used to describe bodily secretions. (Viscus or Viscous)

EXERCISE 3 - MCQs

57. Achilles tendon, also referred to as the calcaneal tendon, is the thickest tendon in the human body. It was named after which one of the following?

    a. A Roman hero
    b. A Viking hero
    c. A Greek hero
    d. A Medieval hero

58. Which one of the following is a potentially life-threatening disease of the adrenal glands associated with insufficient cortisol, named after the physician who first identified it?

    a. Cushing's syndrome
    b. Addison's disease
    c. Parkinson's disease
    d. Alzheimer's disease

59. Which one of the following is a worsening deterioration of the mental faculties, caused by brain degeneration, named after a German neurologist?

    a. Cushing's syndrome
    b. Addison's disease
    c. Parkinson's disease
    d. Alzheimer's disease

60. Virginia Apgar devised a score that proved to be an efficient and quick way to conduct the initial assessment of:

    a. A stroke patient
    b. A newborn child
    c. A toddler
    d. A patient with diabetes

61. Surgeon and neurologist, Charles Bell's name is associated with the paralysis of which cranial nerve?

    a. Optic
    b. Auditory
    c. Glossopharyngeal
    d. Facial

62. Paul Broca, a French anatomist and surgeon, described a condition in stroke patients where they are unable to:

    a. Walk properly
    b. Chew their food
    c. Form complete sentences
    d. Understand basic commands

63. Which one of the following is a series of symptoms brought about by excessively elevated levels of cortisol?

    a. Cushing's syndrome
    b. Addison's disease
    c. Parkinson's disease
    d. Alzheimer's disease

64. The Eustachian tube, also referred to as the auditory tube, serves as a connection between the middle ear and nasopharynx. It is named after:

    a.   An Italian anatomist
    b.   A French surgeon
    c.   A German town
    d.   A Greek myth

65. American surgeon, Henry Heimlich, came up with a technique that can be life-saving in which one of the following conditions?

    a.   Drowning
    b.   Stroke
    c.   Burns
    d.   Choking

66. Homans' sign, named after the American surgeon, John Homans, is indicative of which one of the following conditions?

    a.   Aortic stenosis
    b.   Deep vein thrombosis
    c.   Leg ulcers
    d.   Varicose veins

EXERCISE 4 – TRUE OR FALSE

Set A

67. AIDS: Acquired Immune Deficiency Syndrome ☐

68. ARDS: Acute Renal Distress Syndrome ☐

69. BPH: Benign Prostatic Hypertrophy ☐

70. AF: Atrial Flutter ☐

71. CSF: Cerebrospinal Fluid ☐

72. CNS: Central Nervous Syndrome ☐

73. COPD: Chronic Obstructive Pulmonary Disease ☐

74. CAT scan: Computerized Acute Tomography ☐

75. CVA: Cerebrovascular Accident ☐

76. CXR: Computerized X-ray ☐

77. GERD: Gastroesophageal Reflux Disease ☐

78. EEG: Electroechogram ☐

79. FHR: Fetal Heart Rate ☐

80. ECG: Electrocardiogram ☐

81. ECT: Electrochronic Therapy ☐

82. ET: Endotracheal Tube ☐

83. FB: Foreign Body ☐

84. GI: Gastroischemic ☐

85. ICU: Immediate Care Unit ☐

86. HR: Heart Rate ☐

Set B

87. HRT: Human Replacement Therapy ☐

88. KVO: Keep Vein Open ☐

89. IBS: Irritable Bladder Syndrome ☐

90. IUD: Intrauterine Device ☐

91. IBD: Irritable Bowel Disease ☐

92. NSAID: Non-Steroidal Anti-Inflammatory Drug ☐

93. NG: Nasogastric ☐

94. MRI: Magnetic Respiratory Imaging ☐

95. MS: Multiple Sclerosis ☐

96. MVA: Motor Vehicle Accident ☐

97. PEA: Pulsatile Electrical Activity ☐

98. SZ: Seizure ☐

99. PID: Pelvic Inflammatory Disease ☐

100. PPIs: Proton Positive Inhibitors ☐

101. UA: Urinalysis ☐

102. TAH: Total Aseptic Hysterectomy ☐

103. PT: Prothrombin Time ☐

104. THR: Total Heart Replacement ☐

105. TKR: Total Knee Replacement ☐

106. V/Q SCAN: Ventilation Perfusion Scan ☐

EXERCISE 5 - LABEL THE PICTURE

Use the abbreviations provided in the table below to label the picture.

q.d	STAT	qPM	q12
p.c.	a.c.	q.i.d	b.i.d
qAM	qod	qhs	q2h

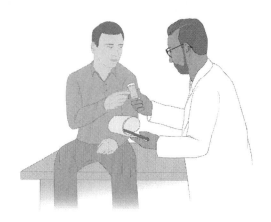

107. Before meals: _____

108. After meals: _____

109. Two times daily: _____

110. Every morning: _____

111. Every day: _____

112. Every other day: _____

113. At bedtime: _____

114. Every 2 hours: _____

115. Strictly every 12 hours: _____

116. Every evening: _____

117. Four times daily: _____

118. Immediately: _____

Pluralizing Medical Terms

EXERCISE 1 - FILL IN THE BLANKS

1. If the singular form of the word ends in an –a suffix, then it is written in the plural form by adding an _____ at the end.

2. If the singular form of the word ends in an –ex suffix or in an –ix suffix, then it is changed into the plural form by turning the ending into _____

3. That said, if the singular word ends in -nx, then the x is removed and changed to _____

4. Still, if the singular form of the words ends only with an -x, then the plural form is created by replacing x with _____ .

5. When it comes to pluralizing singular words ending in –is, the end i is changed into an _____

EXERCISE 2 - MCQs

Choose the correct plural form for the following medical terms.

6. Phalanx:

    a. Phalanxes
    b. Phalanges
    c. Phalanxi

7. Bursa:

    a. Bursae
    b. Bursea
    c. Burses

8. Thorax:

    a. Thoraxi
    b. Thoraxae
    c. Thoraces

9. Femoris:

    a. Femora
    b. Femores
    c. Femorae

10. Iris:

    a. Iritis
    b. Ires
    c. Irides

11. Ganglion:

    a. Gangli
    b. Ganglia
    c. Ganglae

12. Corpus:

    a. Corpit
    b. Corpes
    c. Corpora

13. Viscus:

    a. Visci
    b. Viscera
    c. Viscora

14. Meatus:

    a. Meati
    b. Meates
    c. Meatus

15. Vas:

    a. Vasa
    b. Vasi
    c. Vas

EXERCISE 3 - TRUE OR FALSE

In the following sentences, check if the correct plural form has been used.

16. The aseptic technique is important to eliminate the risk of **infections**. ☐ ☐

17. Due to the leg injury, the patient had to use **crutchs**. ☐ ☐

18. Sometimes, even **placeboes** have remarkable therapeutic effects. ☐ ☐

19. The patient was asked to count backwards by **5s**. ☐ ☐

20. The patient is in his late **50's**. ☐ ☐

UNIT VII

The Structure and Organization of the Body

EXERCISE 1 - MCQs

1. Which one of the following refers to the vertical plane that separates the human body into anterior and posterior halves?

   a. Sagittal Plane
   b. Transverse Plane
   c. Midsagittal Plane
   d. Coronal Plane

2. Which one of the following refers to a vertical plane which separates the left side of the body from the right?

   a. Sagittal Plane
   b. Transverse Plane
   c. Midsagittal Plane
   d. Coronal Plane

3. Which one of the following refers to the vertical plane that separates the body equally into left and right halves?

   a. Sagittal Plane
   b. Transverse Plane
   c. Midsagittal Plane
   d. Coronal Plane

4. Which one of the following refers to a plane parallel to the ground that separates the upper half of the human body from the lower half?

   a. Sagittal Plane
   b. Transverse Plane
   c. Midsagittal Plane
   d. Coronal Plane

EXERCISE 2 - MATCH THE COLUMNS

Set A - Body Positions

	Description	Correct match	Body position
5.	A side-lying position (either left or right) where the knee of one leg is slightly bent		Fowler
6.	Also referred to as the knee-chest position, it is when a patient goes on his knees on an examination table/bed		Sims Position
7.	When the patient is lying face down, and flat on his abdomen		Supine
8.	The patient starts off in the supine position, then, with the thighs apart, the legs are drawn towards the abdomen		Lateral Recumbent
9.	This is when the human body is standing upright, the arms are lying at each side and the palms are faced forward		Erect
10.	A position in which the subject is lying on his back, with the legs at a higher level than the head		Genupectoral
11.	A side-lying position wherein the patient is lying on his left side, but his right thigh and his right knee is pulled up toward his chest		Lithotomy
12.	When the subject is standing upright		Anatomic Position
13.	When the subject is lying flat on his back, facing up		Trendelenburg
14.	The patient lies supine, but the head part of the bed is raised 18 inches and the patient's knees are elevated		Prone

Set B - Four Regions of the Abdomen

	Organs	Correct match	Region
15.	Stomach, pancreas, spleen		RUQ
16.	Appendix		LUQ
17.	Parts of the small and large intestine		RLQ
18.	Liver, gallbladder		LLQ

Set C - The Nine Regions

	Location	Correct match	Region
19.	In the upper left part of the abdomen, specifically under the lower rib cartilage		Region I (Right Hypochondriac Region)
20.	In the abdomen's mid-section, specifically in the middle of the two lumbar regions		Region II (Epigastric Region)
21.	Found in the upper right part of the abdomen, specifically underneath the lower rib cartilage		Region III (Left Hypochondriac Region)
22.	Situated in the mid-left abdominal area		Region IV (Right Lumbar Region)
23.	Found in the lower left abdominal area		Region V (Umbilical Region)
24.	Found in the abdomen's mid-section on the right		Region VI (Left Lumbar Region)
25.	Mid-lower part of the abdomen		Region VII (Right Inguinal Region/ Right Iliac Region)
26.	Situated in the middle of the two hypochondriac regions, specifically in the superior part of the abdomen and below the lower rib cartilage		Region VIII (Hypogastric Region)
27.	Lower right part of the abdomen		Region IX (Left Inguinal Region/Left Iliac Region)

EXERCISE 3 - LABEL THE PICTURE

Name the five regions of the spinal column.

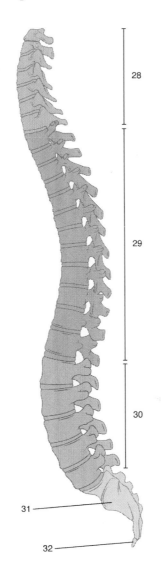

28. _____   31. _____

29. _____   32. _____

30. _____

EXERCISE 4 - MCQs

33. Lymph nodes located around the ear are aptly called:

   a.   Axillary
   b.   Auricular
   c.   Buccal
   d.   Ophthalmic

34. Mucous glands inside the cheeks are referred to as:

   a.   Axillary
   b.   Auricular
   c.   Buccal
   d.   Ophthalmic

35. Big vessels deep in the armpit are termed:

   a.   Axillary
   b.   Auricular
   c.   Buccal
   d.   Ophthalmic

36. The mental nerve innervates the skin around the:

   a.   Head
   b.   Ear
   c.   Chin
   d.   Eye

37. Orbital structures are related to the:

    a.   Head
    b.   Ear
    c.   Chin
    d.   Eye

38. Which body cavity houses the reproductive organs?

    a.   Thoracic
    b.   Abdominal
    c.   Pelvic
    d.   Dorsal

39. The term antebrachial refers to the:

    a.   Inner elbow
    b.   Forearm
    c.   Arm
    d.   Wrist

40. Brachial vessels would be found in the:

    a.   Inner elbow
    b.   Forearm
    c.   Arm
    d.   Wrist

41. Carpal bones would be found in the:

    a.   Inner elbow
    b.   Forearm
    c.   Arm
    d.   Wrist

42. The femoral region corresponds to the:

    a.   Groin
    b.   Thigh
    c.   Knee
    d.   Foot

43. The term inguinal refers to the:

    a.   Groin
    b.   Thigh
    c.   Knee
    d.   Foot

44. Pedal structures would be found in the:

    a.   Groin
    b.   Thigh
    c.   Knee
    d.   Foot

Terminology of Body Systems

EXERCISE 1 - FILL IN THE BLANKS

Set A

1. Angiomas are benign growths made up of small
   _____ .

2. Inflammation of the aorta is known as _____ .

3. Atheroma occurs when damaging _____
   matter accumulates in the inner layer of the arterial walls.

4. A heart specialist is more technically called a
   _____ .

5. _____ is a technique for the aspiration of fluid
   from the pericardial sac.

6. Thrombocytes have a role to play in _____ .

7. Inflammation of the air sacs, found at the end of bronchioles, is
   called _____ .

8. _____ is a device used to monitor and measure the carbon dioxide concentration in exhaled air.

9. Weakening of the larynx, a rare condition that occurs in neonates, is clinically referred to as _____.

10. The clinical term for laugh lines, which run from the nose down to the corner of the mouth, is _____.

11. The pulse oximeter is a device used to monitor the _____ saturation of blood.

Set B

12. _____ refers to hardened deposits in the appendix.

13. Biliary obstruction suggests a blockage in the _____ ducts.

14. Esophageal varices are dilated _____ in the esophagus.

15. Inflammation of the salivary glands is called _____.

16. _____ is an enlargement of the adrenal gland.

17. _____ is a hormone secreted by the pancreas which increases blood glucose levels.

18. The surgical removal of the pancreas is known as _____.

19. In _____, reduced levels of parathyroid hormone in the blood leads to calcium deficiency.

20. Thyrotoxicosis refers to _____ amounts of thyroid hormone.

Set C

21. The term adiposis indicates a disproportionate accumulation of _____ in the body, or in an organ.

22. Dermophytosis denotes a fungal infection of the _____.

23. Anhidrosis is the name of a clinical condition in which the person cannot _____ normally.

24. _____ is the surgical removal of unwanted excess fat beneath the skin.

25. Mycosis is any infection where the causative agent is a _____.

26. Onycholysis is a medical condition that affects the _____.

27. Trichomycosis is a type of infection that affects the _____.

28. The _____ joint is a joint in the arm involving the ulna and humerus bones.

29. _____ is when the spine is curved outward, such as in hunchbacks.

30. The term _____ denotes a smooth muscle tumor that is non-malignant.

31. _____ results from wear and tear of joint cartilage, causing bones to rub against each other.

32. _____ is when the spine is abnormally curved sideways.

33. Synovitis refers to inflammation of the _____.

EXERCISE 2 - MATCH THE COLUMNS

Set A - Nervous System

	Description	Correct match	Root word
34.	Pertaining to the cranium		Mening/ Meningo/ Meningio
35.	Pertains to the cerebellum, the major brain division that governs musculoskeletal movement		Cerebr/ Cerebro/ Cerebri
36.	Concerning the meninges		Neur/Neuri/ Neuro
37.	Pertains to the cerebrum, the major part of the brain that governs feelings, behavior, memory, and thoughts		Crani/ Cranio
38.	Relating to a nerve		Cerebell/ Cerebello

Set B - Sensory System

	Description	Correct match	Medical term
39.	A scratch in the outer layer of the cornea		Dacryocystitis
40.	A surgical procedure wherein an opening is made in the cochlea		Audiometry
41.	Protrusion of the sclera		Corneal abrasion
42.	Infected lacrimal sac/s		Lacrimotomy
43.	The measurement of an individual's sense of hearing, both in terms of sensitivity and range		Conjunctivitis
44.	A surgical incision made into the lacrimal duct		Cochleostomy
45.	When the mucous membrane that lines the eyelid is inflamed		Sclerastasia

Set C - Urinary System

	Description	Correct match	Medical term
46.	A surgical procedure wherein the urinary bladder is attached to the abdominal wall, or to other adjacent structures		Glomerulonephritis
47.	A surgical procedure wherein an opening is created within the ureter, so that the flow of the urine can be diverted away from the bladder		Pyelogram
48.	A condition wherein calcium salts are deposited in the renal parenchyma		Cystopexy
49.	A condition where the glomeruli are inflamed		Nephrocalcinosis
50.	An X-ray inspection of the kidneys, the bladder, and the ureters with the aid of a contrast medium introduced into veins		Ureterostomy

EXERCISE 3 - BUILDING WORDS

Set A - Female Reproductive System

Use the word parts given in the table below to build words that fit the following descriptions.

cele	hystero	colpo	lacto
gram	genic	galacto	itis
cervic	rrhagia	salpingo	

51. A cyst in the mammary gland, that contains milk:

    _____

52. Excessive vaginal bleeding: _____

53. An X-ray exam performed to determine the patency of the uterus and fallopian tubes: _____

54. Inflamed cervix: _____

55. A substance that triggers milk production: _____

Set B - Male Reproductive System

Use the word parts given in the table below to build words that fit the following descriptions.

gen	prostat	a	orchid
spermia	ectomy	andro	itis

56. Inflamed prostate: _____

57. Surgical removal of the testes: _____

58. A hormone which triggers and maintains male characteristics:

_____

59. Absence of sperms in the semen: _____

Answers

UNIT I
UNDERSTANDING MEDICAL TERMS

EXERCISE 1 - FILL IN THE BLANKS

1. root
2. suffixes
3. prefix
4. suffix

EXERCISE 2 - MATCH THE COLUMNS

Set A

5. dys
6. mal
7. emia
8. itis
9. osis
10. pathy

Set B

11. echo
12. electro
13. ectomy
14. gram
15. graph or graphy
16. otomy
17. scopy
18. stomy
19. plasty

UNIT II
ROOT WORDS

EXERCISE 1 - MATCH THE COLUMNS

Set A

1. brain
2. nose
3. eardrum
4. tooth
5. skull
6. eye
7. ear
8. tongue

Set B

9. muscles
10. shoulder
11. arm
12. wrist
13. rib
14. back
15. bones
16. foot

EXERCISE 2 - BUILDING WORDS

17. Cardiology
18. Carditis
19. Echocardiography
20. Echocardiogram
21. Cardiomyopathy
22. Colitis
23. Transesophageal
24. Colectomy
25. Colostomy

EXERCISE 3 - FILL IN THE BLANKS

Set A

26. Acromegaly
27. Axillary
28. blepharoplasty
29. Buccal
30. dermatitis
31. Dorsiflexion
32. gums
33. Laparoscopy
34. unilateral
35. Mammogram

Set B

36. Gynecomastia
37. stomach
38. occipital
39. teeth
40. ophthalmoscope
41. Optometry
42. Oropharyngeal
43. otitis media
44. Pilocystic
45. Podiatry

Set C

46. stethoscope
47. Thoracentesis
48. analgesics
49. bronchoconstrictor
50. carcinogen
51. carcinogenesis
52. Cellulitis

53. cerebrovascular disease
54. cholecystectomy
55. cryosurgery

EXERCISE 4 - TRUE OR FALSE

Set A

56. T
57. T
58. F
59. T
60. F
61. T
62. F
63. T
64. T
65. F

Set B

66. T
67. T
68. F
69. F
70. T
71. F
72. F
73. T
74. F
75. T

Set C

76. F
77. T
78. T

79. F
80. T
81. F
82. T
83. T
84. F
85. F

EXERCISE 5 - MCQs

Set A

86. b
87. c
88. b
89. d
90. c
91. d
92. c
93. d
94. c
95. a

Set B

96. d
97. a
98. c
99. d
100. b
101. a
102. b
103. c
104. b
105. c

EXERCISE 6 - LABEL THE PICTURE

106. Lateral
107. Medial
108. Dorsal
109. Ventral

110. Cranial
111. Caudal
112. Proximal
113. Distal

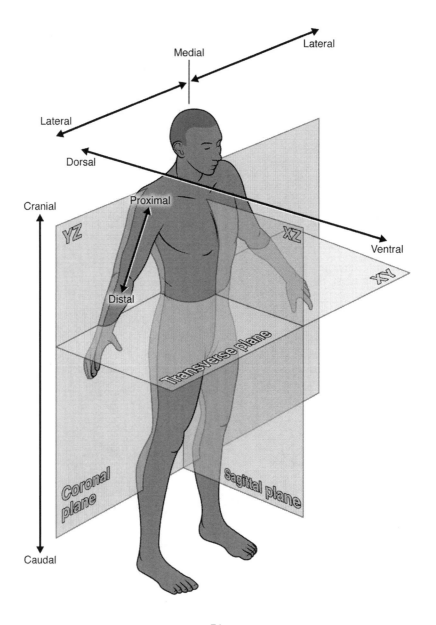

EXERCISE 7 - CROSSWORD

				[114]T					[115]M			
[116]T	H	E	R	M	O	G	R	A	P	H	Y		
				N					O		[117]T	
		[118]D	O	R	S	A					R	
				I		[119]L					A	
[120]U	R	I	N	A	L	Y	S	I	S		C	
				L		P					H	
				E		O					E	
		[121]C		C							O	
	[122]H	Y	P	O	T	H	Y	R	O	I	D	I	S	M
		A		O							T	
		N		M			[123]H	E	M	O	
				Y							M	
											Y	

UNIT III
PRONOUNCING MEDICAL TERMS

EXERCISE 1 - MATCH THE COLUMNS

1. k
2. sk
3. guy
4. n
5. z
6. guh
7. f
8. si
9. j
10. siy

EXERCISE 2 - MCQs

11. b
12. c
13. b
14. a
15. a
16. b
17. b

UNIT IV
PREFIXES AND SUFFIXES

EXERCISE 1 - MATCH THE COLUMNS

Set A

1. auto
2. co/con/com
3. a
4. extra/extro
5. hyp/hypo
6. alb
7. hyper
8. hemi
9. de
10. bi

Set B

11. micro
12. semi

13. idio
14. post
15. intra
16. ultra
17. trans
18. pre
19. syn
20. macro

EXERCISE 2 - MEDICAL ANTONYMS

21. Adduction
22. Tachypnea
23. Exogenous depression
24. Dysthymia
25. Hyperplasia
26. Anterograde amnesia

EXERCISE 3 - MEDICAL SYNONYMS

27. Teeth
28. Nephro
29. Mast/Masto
30. Umbilico

EXERCISE 4 - SYNONYMOUS PREFIXES: PICK THE ODD ONE OUT

31. c
32. b
33. a
34. b

EXERCISE 5 - MCQs

Set A

35. b
36. c
37. b
38. a
39. a

Set B

40. c
41. d
42. a
43. c
44. d
45. d
46. a
47. a
48. c
49. b

EXERCISE 6 - FILL IN THE BLANKS

Set A

50. decibel
51. single/one
52. nullipara
53. primigravida
54. Quadriplegia
55. semicircular
56. tricyclic
57. polydipsia

Set B

58. Arthralgia
59. weakness
60. cystocele
61. Lymphangiectasia
62. hemoglobin
63. sleep
64. Elephantiasis
65. colitis
66. Fecalith
67. anxiety

EXERCISE 7 - TRUE OR FALSE

Set A

68. T
69. F
70. F
71. T
72. F
73. T
74. F
75. F

Set B

76. F
77. T
78. T
79. T
80. F
81. F
82. T
83. T
84. T
85. F

EXERCISE 8 - LABEL THE PICTURE

86. Laryngitis
87. Thyroiditis
88. Bronchitis
89. Carditis
90. Hepatitis
91. Gastritis
92. Cholecystitis
93. Colitis
94. Appendicitis
95. Cystitis

EXERCISE 9 - CROSSWORD

		96 a				97 b		98 s			
	99 e	r	e	100 c	t	i	l	e			
		t		o		l		p			
101 t	h	e	r	a	p	e	u	t	i	c	
		r		g							
		i		u							
	102 c	o	l	l	a	g	e	n	i	c	
		l		a							
103 v	e	n	t	r	i	c	u	l	a	r	
				e							

UNIT V
EPONYMS, HOMONYMS AND MORE

EXERCISE 1 - MATCH THE COLUMNS

Set A

1. Apophysis
2. Agonist
3. Oral
4. Anuresis
5. Epiphysis
6. Core
7. Antagonist
8. Cor
9. Aural
10. Enuresis

Set B

11. Dysphasia
12. Galacturia
13. Diathesis
14. Dyskaryosis
15. Galactorrhea
16. Diastasis
17. Dysphagia
18. Dyskeratosis
19. Diaphysis

Set C

20. DX
21. DTR
22. BKA
23. C&S
24. in vitro
25. CC
26. DNR
27. DVT
28. LUQ

29. FX
30. UTI
31. in vivo
32. npo

Set D

33. @
34. α
35. $\approx$
36. Δ
37. $\uparrow$
38. $\downarrow$
39. ♀
40. ♂
41. <
42. >
43. $\varnothing$

EXERCISE 2 - FILL IN THE BLANKS

Set A

44. Humoral
45. Hypothesis
46. Ileum
47. Lice
48. Malleus
49. Metastasis

Set B

50. Mucus
51. Ostial
52. Perfuse
53. Radicle
54. Resection

81

55. Vesical
56. Viscous

EXERCISE 3 - MCQs

57. c
58. b
59. d
60. b
61. d
62. c
63. a
64. a
65. d
66. b

EXERCISE 4 - TRUE OR FALSE

Set A

67. T
68. F
69. T
70. F
71. T
72. F
73. T
74. F
75. T
76. F
77. T
78. F
79. T
80. T
81. F
82. T
83. T
84. F
85. F
86. T

Set B

87. F
88. T
89. F
90. T
91. F
92. T
93. T
94. F
95. T
96. T
97. F
98. T
99. T
100. F
101. T
102. F
103. T
104. F
105. T
106. T

EXERCISE 5 - LABEL THE PICTURE

107. a.c.
108. p.c.
109. b.i.d
110. qAM
111. q.d
112. qod
113. qhs
114. q2h
115. q12
116. qPM
117. q.i.d
118. STAT

UNIT VI
PLURALIZING MEDICAL TERMS

EXERCISE 1 - FILL IN THE BLANKS

1. e
2. –ices
3. ges
4. ces
5. e

EXERCISE 2 - MCQs

6. b
7. a
8. c
9. a

10. c
11. b
12. c
13. b
14. c
15. a

EXERCISE 3 - TRUE OR FALSE

16. T
17. F
18. F
19. F
20. F

UNIT VII
THE STRUCTURE AND ORGANIZATION OF THE BODY

EXERCISE 1 - MCQs

1. d
2. a
3. c
4. b

9. Anatomic Position
10. Trendelenburg
11. Sims Position
12. Erect
13. Supine
14. Fowler

EXERCISE 2 - MATCH THE COLUMNS

Set A - Body Positions

5. Lateral Recumbent
6. Genupectoral
7. Prone
8. Lithotomy

Set B - Four Regions of the Abdomen

15. LUQ
16. RLQ
17. LLQ
18. RUQ

Set C - The Nine Regions

19. Region III (Left Hypochondriac Region)
20. Region V (Umbilical Region)
21. Region I (Right Hypochondriac Region)
22. Region VI (Left Lumbar Region)
23. Region IX (Left Inguinal Region/Left Iliac Region)
24. Region IV (Right Lumbar Region)
25. Region VIII (Hypogastric Region)
26. Region II (Epigastric Region)
27. Region VII (Right Inguinal Region/Right Iliac Region)

EXERCISE 3 - LABEL THE PICTURE

28. Cervical
29. Thoracic
30. Lumbar
31. Sacral
32. Coccygeal

EXERCISE 4 - MCQs

33. b
34. c
35. a
36. c
37. d
38. c
39. b
40. c
41. d
42. b
43. a
44. d

UNIT VIII
TERMINOLOGY OF BODY SYSTEMS

EXERCISE 1 - FILL IN THE BLANKS

Set A

1. blood vessels
2. aortitis
3. fatty
4. cardiologist
5. Pericardiocentesis
6. clotting/blood clotting
7. alveolitis
8. Capnometer
9. laryngomalacia
10. Nasolabial folds
11. oxygen

Set B

12. Appendicolith
13. bile
14. veins
15. sialadenitis
16. Adrenomegaly

17. Glucagon
18. pancreatectomy
19. hypoparathyroidism
20. excessive/increased

Set C

21. fat
22. skin
23. sweat/perspire
24. Liposuction
25. fungus
26. nails
27. hair
28. humeroulnar
29. Kyphosis
30. leiomyoma
31. Osteoarthritis
32. Scoliosis
33. synovial membrane

EXERCISE 2 - MATCH THE COLUMNS

Set A - Nervous System

34. Crani/Cranio
35. Cerebell/Cerebello
36. Mening/Meningo/ Meningio
37. Cerebr/Cerebro/Cerebri
38. Neur/Neuri/Neuro

Set B - Sensory System

39. Corneal abrasion
40. Cochleostomy

41. Sclerastasia
42. Dacryocystitis
43. Audiometry
44. Lacrimotomy
45. Conjunctivitis

Set C - Urinary System

46. Cystopexy
47. Ureterostomy
48. Nephrocalcinosis
49. Glomerulonephritis
50. Pyelogram

EXERCISE 3 - BUILDING WORDS

Set A - Female Reproductive System

51. galactocele
52. colporrhagia
53. hysterosalpingogram
54. cervicitis
55. lactogenic

Set B - Male Reproductive System

56. prostatitis
57. orchidectomy
58. androgen
59. aspermia

JOIN OUR COMMUNITY

Medical Creations® is an educational company focused on providing study tools for Healthcare students.

You can find all of our products at this link: **www.medicalcreations.net**

If you have any questions or concerns please contact us: **hello@medicalcreations.net**

We want to be as close as possible to our customers, that's why we are active on all the main Social Media platforms.

You can find us here:

      Facebook **www.facebook.com/medicalcreations**
      Instagram **www.instagram.com/medicalcreationsofficial**
      Pinterest **www.pinterest.com/medicalcreations**
      Website: **www.medicalcreations.net**

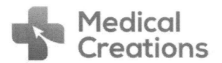

CHECK OUT OUR OTHER BOOKS

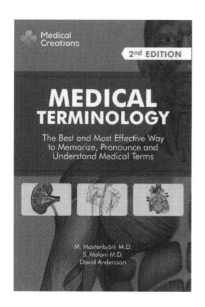

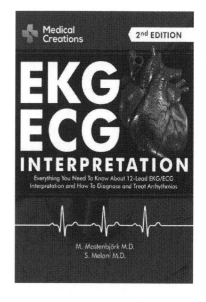

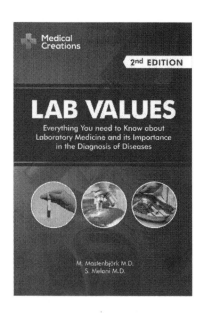

Lab Values: Everything You Need to Know about Laboratory Medicine and its Importance in the Diagnosis of Diseases

Fluids and Electrolytes: A Thorough Guide covering Fluids, Electrolytes and Acid-Base Balance of the Human Body

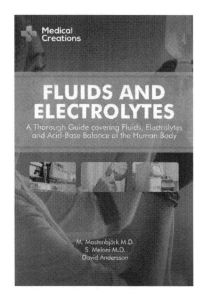

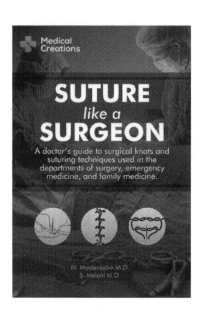

Suture like a Surgeon:
A Doctor's Guide to Surgical Knots
and Suturing Techniques used in the
Departments of Surgery, Emergency
Medicine, and Family Medicine

**Advanced Cardiovascular Life
Support (ACLS)**
Provider Manual -
A Comprehensive Guide
Covering the Latest Guidelines

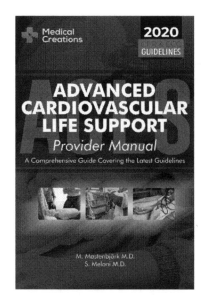

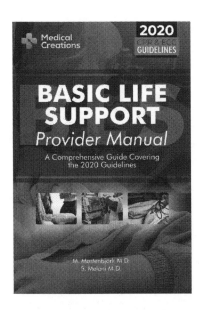

Basic Life Support
Provider Manual -
A Comprehensive Guide
Covering the Latest Guidelines

Pharmacology
Review - A Comprehensive
Reference Guide for
Medical, Nursing, and
Paramedic Students

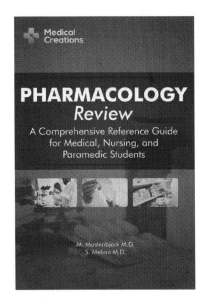

Medical Creations Suture Practice Kit with Suturing Video Series
by Board-Certified Surgeon and Ebook Training Guide

SUTURE LIKE A SURGEON PRACTICE KIT

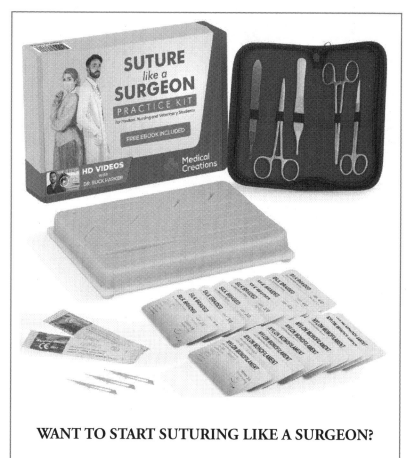

WANT TO START SUTURING LIKE A SURGEON?

Our Suture Practice Kit contains all of the tools
you need to start practicing.

Phlebotomy Practice Kit with Ebook Training Guide -
Complete IV Practice Kit for Venipuncture

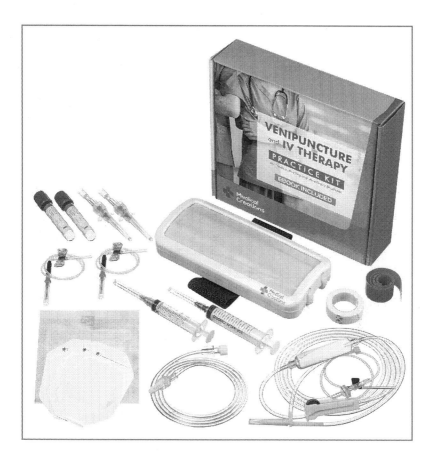

Learn more on our website:
www.medicalcreations.net

NOTES

NOTES

NOTES